TEAM LEADERS AND SUPERVISORS

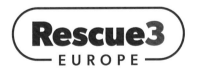

www.rescue3europe.com

ISBN: 978-1-915623-16-4

Authors: Keith Dudhnath and Jonathan Gorman, with additional contributions from Kitty Davies.

Photographs: Devon and Somerset Fire and Rescue Service, Eurosafe, IPH Hitzkirch, Karri Kivenen, Kayak Metavasi – Rescue 3 Greece, Gregor Nigg, and Magnús Stefan Sigurdsson.

Safety Notice

This Rescue 3 Europe manual is a basic text to be used in conjunction with Rescue 3 classes taught by instructors certified by Rescue 3. Utilisation of this material without certified instruction may be hazardous to life and limb.

CONTENTS

RESCUE 3 CONTACT DETAILS

For a list of course providers in your area, please contact Rescue 3 Europe.

RESCUE 3 EUROPE LTD
The Malthouse
Regent Street
Llangollen
Denbighshire
LL20 8HS

Tel +44 (0) 1978 869 069
Web site www.rescue3europe.com
Email info@rescue3europe.com

RESCUE 3 INTERNATIONAL
11084A Jeff Brian Lane
PO Box 1050
Wilton
California 95693
USA

Tel +1 916 687 6556
Fax +1 888 457 3727
Web site www.rescue3.com
Email info@rescue3.com

ABOUT RESCUE 3 EUROPE

Rescue 3 Europe develops state of the art technical rescue courses, providing internationally recognised accreditation for organisations and individuals operating in high risk environments.

As an international accrediting body, Rescue 3 provide up to date best practice guidance that is constantly evolving in line with new research and testing. All changes and developments of Rescue 3 courses go through a process of peer review and oversight by a steering committee made up of industry experts from all over the world.

Rescue 3 training providers deliver courses worldwide, in multiple disciplines, including: water, rope, boat, ice and confined space rescue. Our large suite of courses have been adopted by mountain rescue teams, wind turbine operators, fire and rescue services, ambulance teams, utilities providers, and military personnel.

Within each discipline, Rescue 3 accredited courses cover every level of operations, whether this is at an awareness level, avoiding risks and applying simple safe systems of work; or at more advanced levels where practitioners must acquire high levels of personal skills and understanding to access and navigate difficult environments.

For over four decades Rescue 3 has provided the standard for technical rescue training, offering guidance and support for maintaining best practice.

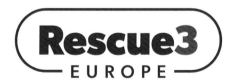

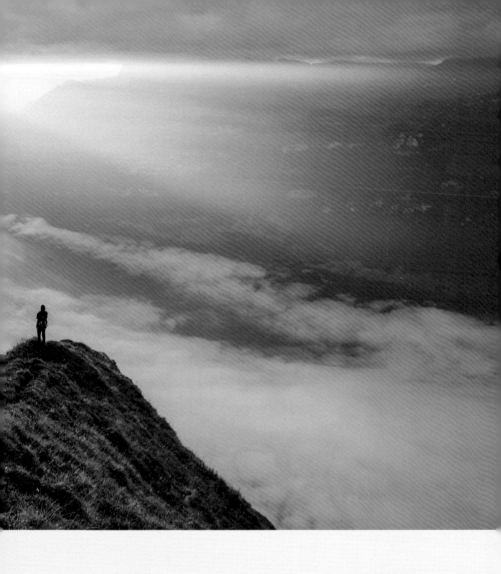

ABOUT THE
TEAM LEADER

WHAT IS A TEAM LEADER?

A team leader is in charge of a technical rescue team. The team leader has at least the same level of technical training as their colleagues. Depending on their organisation, they may have a higher level of technical training.

In addition, the team leader also has training and experience in their supervisory role. The team leader provides a link between operational rescuers and management.

KEY DUTIES OF A TEAM LEADER

▷ Supervising a team of rescuers throughout the operation

▷ Understanding and applying pre-plans and risk assessments

▷ Incident size-up

▷ Selecting a plan of action

▷ Performing team briefings and debriefings

▷ Team welfare (if there isn't a separate welfare officer)

▷ Liaising between operational rescuers and management

▷ Post-incident paperwork and reporting

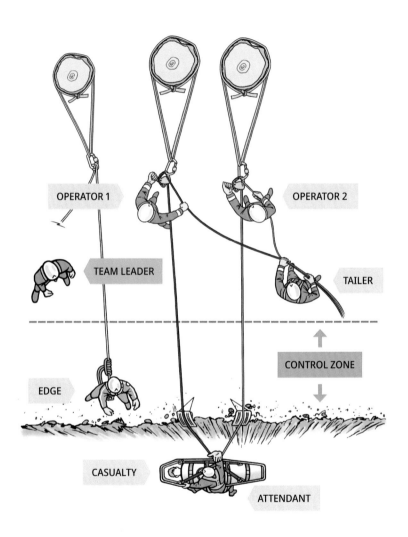

OPERATOR 1

OPERATOR 2

TEAM LEADER

TAILER

CONTROL ZONE

EDGE

CASUALTY

ATTENDANT

Team leader of a rope rescue team

LEADERSHIP STYLES

Psychologist Dr Kurt Lewin's 1939 study identified three key leadership styles. Team leaders should understand the strengths and weaknesses of each style, and draw from them to get the best from their team.

AUTHORITARIAN

The authoritarian style is also known as the autocratic style. The team leader gives clear commands of what is to be done, how it's to be done, and when it's to be done.

This style may be suited to formal command structures, and operational circumstances that require swift and decisive actions.

However, the authoritarian style can miss out on key input from team members. In some circumstances, it may lead to a perception of the team leader being dictatorial, or even creating conflict within the team.

PARTICIPATIVE

The participative style is also known as the democratic style. The team leader gives guidance, but also seeks input from team members. The team leader will collate and assess this input, before presenting their final decision.

This style may be suited to pre-planning and post-incident evaluation. However, during the time pressure of an active rescue, it may not be possible or practical to seek detailed input from all team members.

DELEGATIVE

The delegative style is also known as the laissez-faire style. The team leader is hands-off, offering little guidance, and leaving the final decision up to the team members.

The lack of structure with the delegative style can be problematic for most rescue teams. However, it may be productive in the rare circumstance of an elite team of experts who are highly self-motivated and highly skilled.

In reality, a situational approach will work best for team leaders. The team leader should apply components of each leadership style that best fits the task and circumstances.

A team leader may get the best from their team by taking a participative approach – seeking input from their knowledgeable and skilled colleagues, before making a final decision themselves. Such an approach works brilliantly during pre-planning and post-incident evaluation.

However, during a complex operation, where it becomes necessary to adjust the plan, the team leader may not have the luxury of being able to discuss all the options at length with the team members. A more authoritarian approach may be necessary at that time – whilst still being open for any team member to raise safety-critical concerns.

BEHAVIOURAL ATTRIBUTES OF TEAM MEMBERS

An effective team leader should understand the behavioural attributes of their team members, to get the best from their team and assign tasks most productively.

An individual team member may fulfil multiple behavioural attributes at once. Whilst a team may not require all the identified behavioural attributes at all times, an effective team leader will recognise and make use of the strengths of their team members, and mitigate their weaknesses.

The research of Dr Meredith Belbin refers to these attributes as 'team roles', but this should not be confused with operational team roles (eg upstream spotter, downstream safety in water rescue, or edge, tailer, attendant in rope rescue).

Belbin's 9 team roles/behavioural attributes are:

CO-ORDINATOR

A good candidate for a team leader. Identifies and focuses the team's objectives. Delegates work.

May be perceived as manipulative, if not in a team leader role.

RESOURCE INVESTIGATOR

Inquisitive, finds new ideas to bring to the team.

May be over-optimistic, or lose interest after initial enthusiasm.

TEAMWORKER

Versatile, which can be used to complete many tasks. Brings cohesion to the team through co-operation and diplomacy.

May avoid confrontation or be indecisive.

PLANT

Creative, and may have unconventional solutions to problems. Named because the initial research 'planted' such a person in a team for a creative spark.

May ignore details, or be absent-minded.

MONITOR EVALUATOR

Logical and impartial, judging all options dispassionately.

May be overly critical, or slow to decide.

SPECIALIST

Has in-depth knowledge of a key area.

May only have a narrow focus, or concentrate too much on small details.

SHAPER

Drives and motivates the team, ensuring they don't lose focus, or get waylaid by obstacles.

May be blunt or in their attempts to get things done.

IMPLEMENTER

Practical, reliable, efficient and organised.

May be inflexible or slow to accept new possibilities.

COMPLETER FINISHER

Meticulous checking. Seeks out errors to correct.

May be reluctant to delegate, or take their perfectionism to extremes.

TEAM DEVELOPMENT

For a team to develop as an effective group, they go through a number of stages. Team leaders should be aware of these stages, to better understand why there are particular dynamics within their team. Dr Bruce Tuckman defined these stages as:

FORMING

The team is newly formed, perhaps with people who have not met before, or there are new recruits to the team. Team members may display a mix of excitement and trepidation or uncertainty.

The team leader should define clear structure, direction, goals and roles.

STORMING

Elements of 'stormy' conflict appear in the storming stage, as team members discover differences, frustrations or concerns. Such frustrations may be about the pace of progress, or the processes involved.

The team leader should seek to understand the frustrations of team members, address any issues raised, find solutions, and/or manage expectations as appropriate.

NORMING

The norming stage bridges the gap between the expectations of the forming stage, and any reality checks in the storming stage. Team members increase their understanding and acceptance of other team members and the team's circumstance. They can resolve most conflict with minimal input from the team leader.

Team leaders should provide support and guidance, reaffirming the team's goals and practices. Team leaders can also take the opportunity to re-evaluate these goals and practices during the norming stage.

PERFORMING

The team is working like a well-oiled machine. Team members are satisfied by the team's effectiveness. They understand and appreciate the strengths and weaknesses of themselves and their fellow team members.

Team leaders should monitor and support the team and its members during the performing stage, and celebrate key successes. Team leaders should also be aware of changes in circumstance or personnel which may shift the team to an earlier stage of development.

ADJOURNING

The adjourning stage only applies if a team is coming to an end, or if there are significant changes in personnel (eg retirement of key team members). The team and its members may experience conflicting feelings, including anxiety about the future, sadness, and/or satisfaction about the accomplishments of the team. This may lead to a loss of focus and productivity.

A team leader steering a team through a successful adjourning stage will ensure that all required tasks are completed. They will also evaluate the work of the team, and identify lessons learned, which can be applied in future roles or with future team members. Finally, they will enact a form of closing celebration, recognising and acknowledging the individual and team successes and accomplishments. This will serve as a formal end for the team, or retiring/leaving personnel.

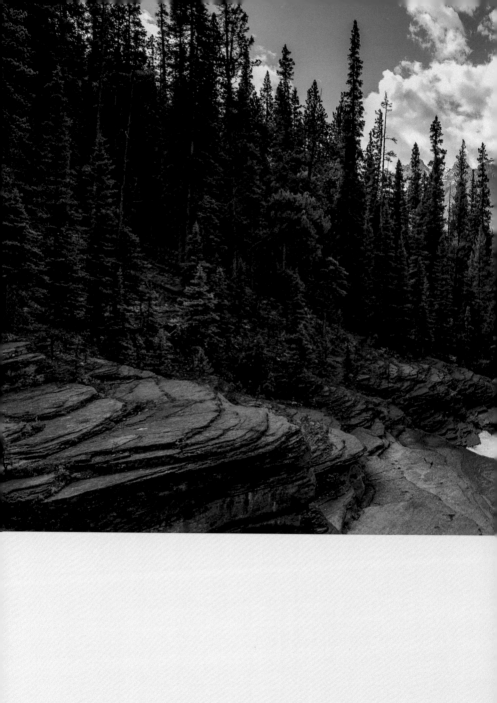

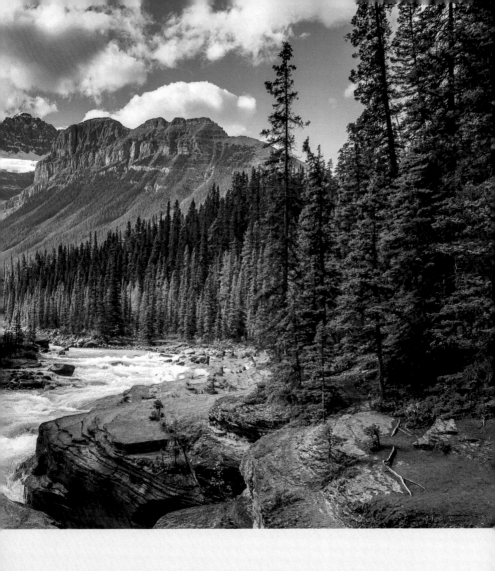

PRE-INCIDENT

LEGISLATION, DOCUMENTATION AND GUIDANCE

Rescue team leaders attending rescue incidents should have an understanding of relevant local, regional and national legislation, documentation and guidance and how they affect their rescue team.

Legislation exists at multinational, national and regional level, that defines systems that should be in place when working and performing rescues in high risk environments.

This manual covers the general principles, which are the same the world over. However, rescue teams should always refer to their applicable local legislation.

Applicable legislation may exist as both generic safety at work legislation (such as the European Framework Directive on Safety and Health at Work, or the USA's Occupational Safety and Health Act 1970), or task-specific legislation (such as the UK's Work at Height Regulations 2005, Arbowet and Arbobesluit in the Netherlands, or Canada's Occupational Health and Safety Regulations).

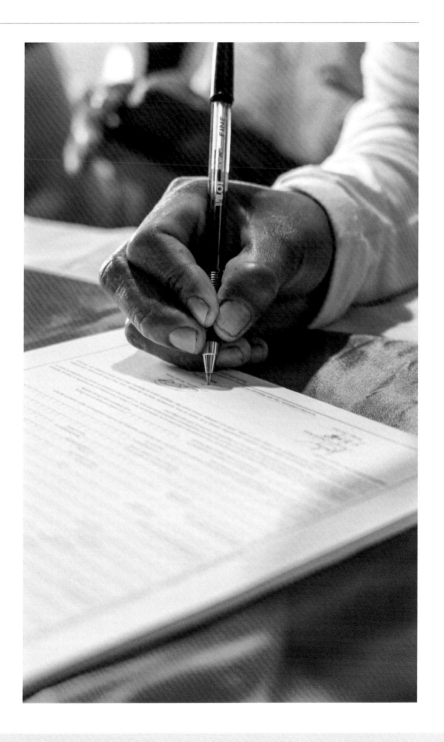

TEAM TYPING

Team leaders should have an understanding of team types used in their area/country and their capability.

Team typing may define either a minimum or an optimum composition of a team.

Team typing will define:

▷ Number of members

▷ Training competencies for operation (eg RRO, SRT, SFRBO)

▷ Additional training (eg first aid/medical, driving)

▷ Logistics capabilities (eg availability, self-sufficiency, financing)

▷ PPE requirements for each member

▷ Technical and team equipment, including:

  › Operational equipment

  › Transport/vehicle details

  › Communications equipment/details

  › Medical and decontamination equipment

  › Navigation equipment/details

  › Lighting and zoning equipment

Example team types are shown for water and boat teams (from page 23), and rope teams (from page 41).

TEAM TYPING - WATER AND BOAT

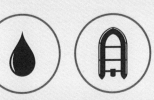

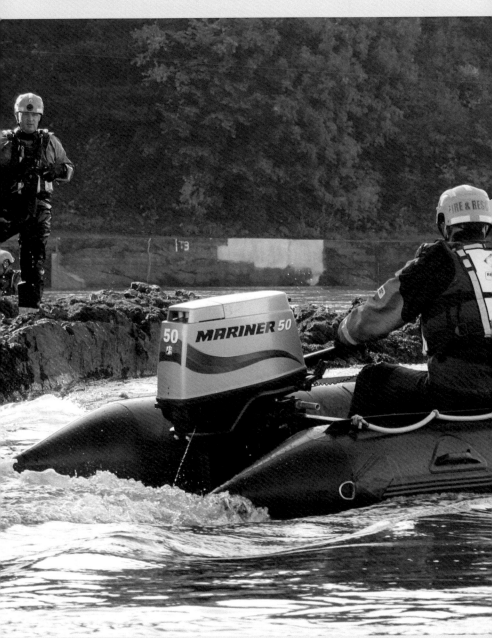

DEFRA WATER TEAM TYPE DESCRIPTIONS

	TEAM TYPE	CAPABILITY
A	Amalgamated Team	▷ Known as A–B for powerboats and A–C for mixed teams ▷ Not pre-declared, but established during the incident ▷ Eg embedding a health care professional, police officer or animal rescue specialist in a B or C team
B	Water Rescue Boat Team	▷ Technical water rescue ▷ Search operations within water environment ▷ Powered boat rescue operations ▷ In-water operations ▷ Flood response
C	Water Rescue Technician Team	▷ Technical water rescue ▷ Search operations within water environment ▷ Non-powered boat rescue operations ▷ In-water operations ▷ Flood response
D	Water Rescue First Responder Team	▷ Support operations ▷ Limited in-water operations ▷ Bank-based safety ▷ Flood response

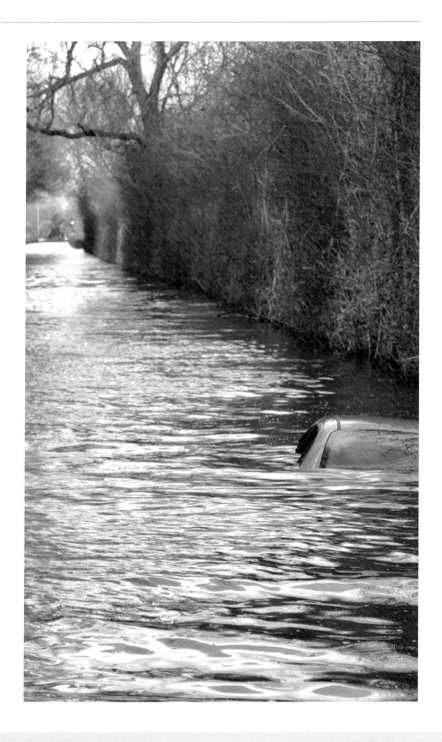

DEFRA TYPE B – WATER RESCUE BOAT TEAM

CAPABILITY

- Technical water rescue
- Search operations within the water environment.
- Power boat rescue operations
- In water operations
- Flood response

LOGISTICS (MINIMUM REQUIREMENTS)

- Be available 24 hours a day
- Facility for financing supplies and consumables when mobile or on scene (eg credit card or Team Manager)
- Team to be sustainable with rations for 10 hours.
- Team to be available for up to 4 days on scene.

TEAM STRUCTURE (MINIMUM 7 PERSONS)

- 1 welfare and liaison officer
- 1 team leader
- 5 team members
- Welfare and liaison officer is for support and welfare considerations at protracted incidents not for tactical command as required by the agency.

COMPETENCIES OF PERSONNEL (MINIMUM NUMBER REQUIRED)

- Module 1 Water Awareness – All
- Module 3 Water Rescue Technicians (6)
- Module 4 Water Rescue Boat Operators (4)
- First Aid Qualified (6). Minimum 2 with advanced training, including water-specific medical considerations.
- Update of training – current and refreshed within the previous 3 year period. Boat and in water skills within a 12 monthly period.

INCIDENT COMMAND SYSTEM

- All team members to be trained to the current ICS in operation for flood incidents.

TEAM TYPE B – EQUIPMENT

TRANSPORT

> Vehicle(s) suitable to carry personnel and equipment.

BOAT

> Minimum capacity to drive upstream against 10mph flow whilst carrying 6 persons.
> Prop guarded.
> Ancillary equipment:
>> anchor
>> fuel containers
>> lifelines
>> D rings for tethers
>> paddles
>> suitable transportation system

COMMUNICATIONS

> Handheld communications for all team members, spare batteries and charger. Waterproofed.
> Mobile phone with team leader and manager. Waterproofed.

PPE

> Full PPE for all team members, and redundancy
> Drysuit
> Buoyancy aid
> Helmet
> Footwear
> Gloves
> Knife
> Whistle
> Personal lighting
> Thermal undersuit x 2

MEDICAL

▷ Basic Life Support First Aid Pack – dry bag
▷ Oxygen cylinder x 2 and resuscitation equipment – dry bag
▷ Spinal long board
▷ Blankets
▷ Basket stretcher

TECHNICAL EQUIPMENT

▷ Set of technical rescue equipment including ropes and hardware. Suitable container.
▷ Search equipment including lighting, marker boards, mapping, aides-mémoire.
▷ Throw bags x 8
▷ Scene lighting
▷ Search lighting
▷ Hand tool kit.
▷ Wading Poles

DECONTAMINATION

▷ Anti-bacterial hand gel
▷ Anti-bacterial face wipes
▷ Anti-bacterial equipment spray
▷ Full cleaning facilities available at base station

TESTING

▷ All equipment should be suitably tested, maintained and certified in accordance with manufacturers' guidelines.

NAVIGATION

▷ Handheld GPS system with street mapping facility.

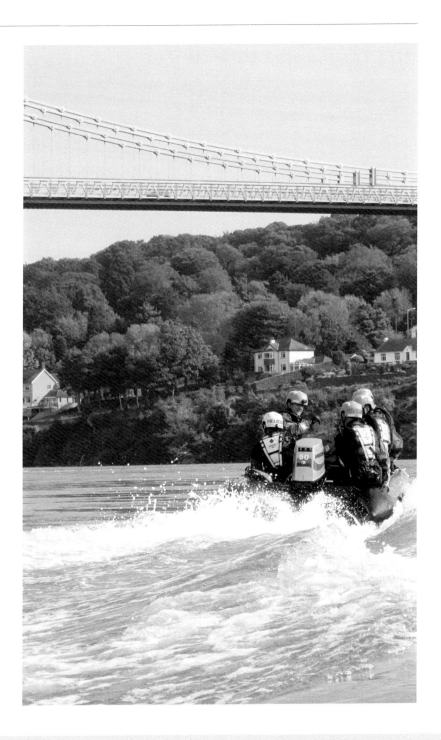

TYPE C – WATER RESCUE TECHNICIAN TEAM

CAPABILITY

- Technical water rescue
- Search operations within the water environment.
- In-water operations
- Non-powered boat operations
- Flood response

LOGISTICS (MINIMUM REQUIREMENTS)

- Be available 24 hours a day
- Facility for financing supplies and consumables when mobile or on scene (eg credit card or Team Manager)
- Team to be sustainable with rations for 10 hours.
- Team to be available for up to 4 days on scene.

TEAM STRUCTURE (MINIMUM 7 PERSONS)

- 1 welfare and liaison officer
- 1 team leader
- 5 team members
- Welfare and liaison officer is for support and welfare considerations at protracted incidents not for tactical command as required by the agency.

COMPETENCIES OF PERSONNEL (MINIMUM NUMBER REQUIRED)

- Module 1 Water Awareness – All
- Module 3 Water Rescue Technicians (6)
- First Aid Qualified (6). Minimum 2 with advanced training, inc. water-specific medical considerations.
- Update of training – current and refreshed within the previous 3 year period. Boat and in water skills within a 12 monthly period.

INCIDENT COMMAND SYSTEM

- All team members to be trained to the current ICS in operation for flood incidents.

TEAM TYPE C – EQUIPMENT

TRANSPORT

- Vehicle(s) suitable to carry personnel and equipment.

BOAT

- Minimum 6 persons capacity for tethering operations or basic paddle boat handling.
- Suitable for wading/paddling rescue of persons without unduly getting the casualties wet.
- Ancillary equipment:
  - anchor
  - fuel containers
  - lifelines
  - D rings for tethers
  - paddles
  - suitable transportation system

COMMUNICATIONS

- Handheld communications for all team members, spare batteries and charger. Waterproofed.
- Mobile phone with team leader and manager. Waterproofed.

PPE

- Full PPE for all team members, and redundancy
- Drysuit
- Buoyancy aid
- Helmet
- Footwear
- Gloves
- Knife
- Whistle
- Personal lighting
- Thermal undersuit x 2

MEDICAL

▷ Basic Life Support First Aid Pack – dry bag
▷ Oxygen cylinder x 2 and resuscitation equipment – dry bag
▷ Spinal long board
▷ Blankets
▷ Basket stretcher

TECHNICAL EQUIPMENT

▷ Set of technical rescue equipment including ropes and hardware. Suitable container.
▷ Throw bags x 8.
▷ Scene lighting.
▷ Search lighting.
▷ Hand tool kit.
▷ Wading poles.
▷ Casualty lifejackets.

DECONTAMINATION

▷ Anti-bacterial hand gel
▷ Anti-bacterial face wipes
▷ Anti-bacterial equipment spray
▷ Full cleaning facilities available at base station

TESTING

▷ All equipment should be suitably tested, maintained and certified in accordance with manufacturers' guidelines.

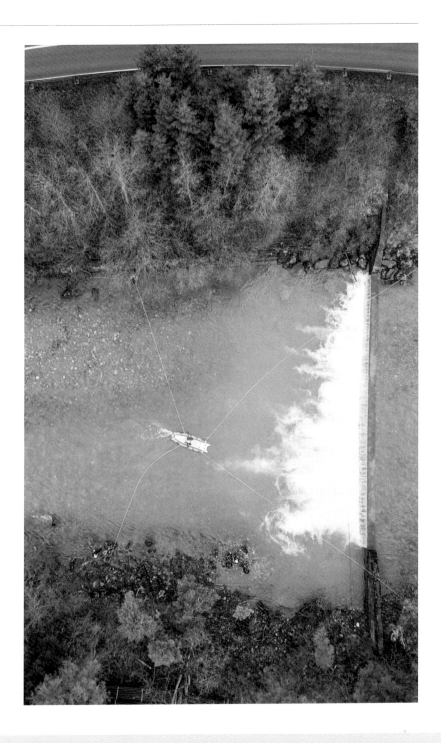

TYPE D – WATER FIRST RESPONDER TEAM

CAPABILITY

▷ Support operations
▷ Bank based safety
▷ Flood response
▷ Wading rescues

LOGISTICS (MINIMUM REQUIREMENTS)

▷ Be available 24 hours a day
▷ Facility for financing supplies and consumables when mobile or on scene (eg credit card or Team Manager)
▷ Team to be sustainable with rations for 10 hours.
▷ Team to be available for up to 4 days on scene.

TEAM STRUCTURE (MINIMUM 4 PERSONS)

▷ 1 team leader
▷ 3 team members
▷ Welfare and liaison officer is for support and welfare considerations at protracted incidents not for tactical command as required by the agency.

COMPETENCIES OF PERSONNEL (MINIMUM NUMBER REQUIRED)

▷ Module 1 Water Awareness (4)
▷ Module 2 Water First Responder (4)
▷ First Aid Qualified (4).
▷ Update of training – current and refreshed within the previous 3 year period.

INCIDENT COMMAND SYSTEM

▷ All team members to be trained to the current ICS in operation for flood incidents.

TEAM TYPE D – EQUIPMENT

TRANSPORT

- Vehicle(s) suitable to carry personnel and equipment.

BOAT (OPTIONAL)

- Minimum 6 persons capacity, suitable for wading rescues of persons without unduly getting the casualties wet.
- Suitable transportation system.

COMMUNICATIONS

- Handheld communications for all team members, spare batteries and charger. Waterproofed.
- Mobile phone with team leader and manager. Waterproofed.

PPE

- Full PPE for all team members, and redundancy
- Drysuit
- Buoyancy aid
- Helmet
- Footwear
- Gloves
- Knife
- Whistle
- Personal lighting
- Thermal undersuit x 2

MEDICAL

- Basic Life Support First Aid Pack
- Oxygen cylinder x 2 and resuscitation equipment
- Blankets

TECHNICAL EQUIPMENT

▷ Throwbags x 5
▷ Scene lighting
▷ Hand tool kit
▷ Wading poles

DECONTAMINATION

▷ Anti-bacterial hand gel
▷ Anti-bacterial face wipes
▷ Anti-bacterial equipment spray
▷ Full cleaning facilities available at base station

TESTING

▷ All equipment should be suitably tested, maintained and certified in accordance with manufacturers' guidelines.

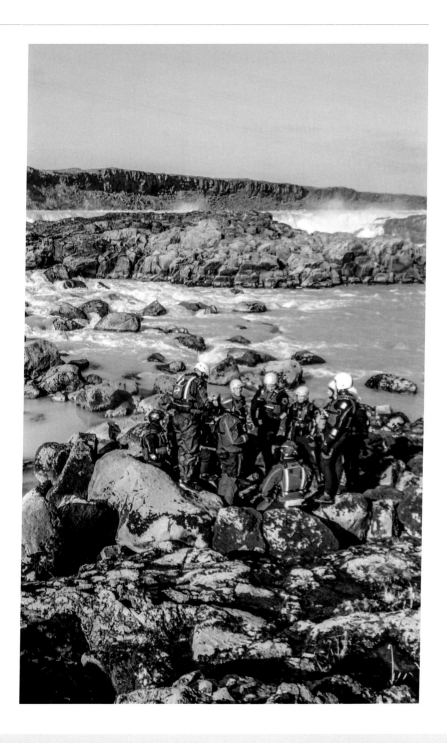

FEMA TYPE 3 SWIFTWATER/FLOOD SEARCH AND RESCUE TEAM

OVERALL FUNCTION

The Swiftwater/Flood SAR Team:

1. Searches for and rescues individuals who may be injured or otherwise in need of medical attention
2. Provides emergency medical care, including Basic Life Support (BLS)
3. Provides animal rescue
4. Transports humans and animals to the nearest location for secondary land or air transport
5. Provides shore-based and boat-based water rescue for humans and animals
6. Supports helicopter rescue operations and urban SAR in water environments for humans and animals
7. Operates in environments with or without infrastructure, including environments with compromised access to roadways, utilities, transportation and medical facilities, and with limited access to shelter, food and water

OPERATIONAL CAPABILITY

1. Performs the following water operations in water with a current of 1 knot or greater:
   > Paddle and powerboat operations
   > Offensive water rescue
   > Flood response operations
2. Performs first aid, including cardiopulmonary resuscitation (CPR) and automated external defibrillator (AED) use
3. Requests rope rescue and aviation resources as necessary
4. Operates in HAZMAT-contaminated environments
5. Manages search operations
6. Provides medical care, including BLS
7. Performs low-angle rope rescue
8. Demonstrates self-sufficiency as the operational environment demands

PERSONNEL PER TEAM (MIMIMUM 6 PEOPLE)

- 1 x NIMS Swiftwater/Flood SAR Team Leader
- 2 x NIMS Swiftwater/Flood SAR Technician – Boat Operator
- 2 x NIMS Swiftwater/Flood SAR Technician – Boat Bowman
- 1 x NIMS Swiftwater/Flood SAR Technician
- 1 of the team members should also hold a NIMS Type 1 EMT qualification.
- 1 of the team members should also have logistics management knowledge.

RECOVERY EQUIPMENT PER RESCUE BOAT

- 3 x Throw bag
- Throwable flotation device
- Vessel support kit
- Paddles
- Swimmer rescue board

DECONTAMINATION EQUIPMENT PER TEAM

- 2 x 25-foot (7.5m) garden hose
- Garden hose wye valve
- Decontamination equipment kit including, for example:
  - 2.5-gallon pressure sprayer
  - 5-gallon bucket
  - Soap and bleach solution
  - 40-gallon plastic work box
  - 110-volt submersible pump
  - 110-volt power washer

GROUND TRANSPORTATION EQUIPMENT PER TEAM

- Vehicle(s) and trailer(s) capable of hauling personnel, equipment and boats
- Tie-downs and strapping

COMMUNICATIONS EQUIPMENT PER TEAM MEMBER

- Two-way handheld radio
- Mobile phone (waterproof)
- Chargers for devices

COMMUNICATIONS EQUIPMENT PER BOAT CREW

- Marine band radio (portable/waterproof)
- Portable radio with ground-to-air capability
- Handheld GPS unit

PERSONAL PROTECTIVE EQUIPMENT (PPE) PER TEAM MEMBER

- Swiftwater/flood SAR helmet
- Headlamp and batteries
- Eye and hearing protection
- Respiratory protection
- Uniform/protective clothing
- Gloves
- Footwear
- Dry suit
- Appropriate Personal Flotation Device (PFD)
- Deployment/travel pack
- Personal medical kit
- Survival kit
- Other necessary field packs or gear

RESCUE EQUIPMENT PER TEAM

- Powered saw and appropriate fuel
- Rope rescue kit
- Pole for reaching (pike or equivalent)
- Assorted hand tools, including Halligan bar, 8-lb. flathead ax, 10-lb. sledgehammer, hammers, drills and saws

RESCUE BOAT EQUIPMENT PER TEAM

- Vehicle(s) and trailer(s) capable of hauling personnel, equipment Inflatable rescue boat or watercraft appropriate for type of water, equipped with supplies and fuel

TEAM TYPING - ROPE

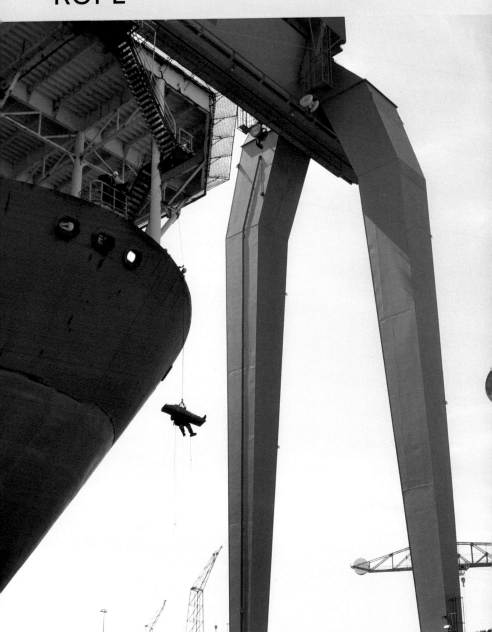

NFCC ROPE TEAM TYPE DESCRIPTIONS

	TEAM TYPE	CAPABILITY
1	Safe Work at Height Team	▷ Knowledge, skills and equipment necessary to work safely at height in order to carry out operational duties. ▷ Knowledge of and skills relevant to the systems, practices and equipment required to implement safe systems of work when work restraint and fall arrest are required.
2	Twin-rope Access and Stabilisation Team	▷ Knowledge, skills and equipment necessary to access and stabilise casualties at height when lowering or raising in a vertical situation is required.
3	Technical Rope Rescue Team	▷ Knowledge of and skills relevant to the systems, practices and equipment required to initiate complex rope access and rescue systems, including: ▷ Work in suspension, lowering and descending ▷ Raising, ascending, traversing structures and landscapes both vertically and non-vertically by deviation or cableway ▷ Full technical rope rescue capability.
LACE	USAR – Line Access Casualty Extrication Team	▷ USAR-trained personnel operating specific USAR wire rope-based systems and ability to create artificial rated anchors (eye bolts).

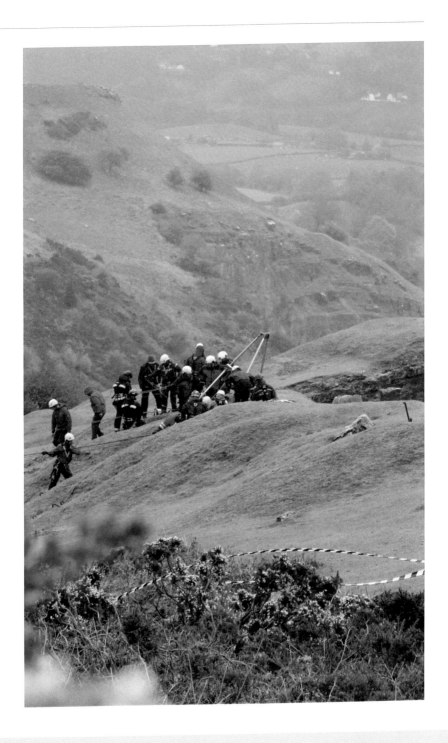

TYPE 3 – ROPE RESCUE TEAM

CAPABILITY

▷ Knowledge, skills and equipment necessary to rig complex rope access and rescue systems, to include rope access work in suspension, lowering, descending, raising, ascending and traversing non-vertically by deviation/cableway.

LOGISTICS (MINIMUM REQUIREMENTS FOR RESPONSE OUTSIDE SERVICE AREA)

▷ Be available 24 hours a day
▷ Facility for financing supplies and consumables when mobile or on scene (eg credit card or Team Manager)
▷ Team to be sustainable with rations for 24 hours.
▷ Team to be available for up to 4 days on scene.

TEAM STRUCTURE (MINIMUM 5 PEOPLE)

▷ 5 team members, including team leader.
▷ 1 welfare and liaison officer
▷ Welfare and liaison officer is for support and welfare considerations at protracted incidents not for tactical command as required by the agency.

COMPETENCIES OF PERSONNEL (MINIMUM NUMBER REQUIRED)

▷ Safe work at height – All
▷ Level 3 technician – All
▷ First Aid Qualified – All
▷ Up-to-date training refers to current training that has been refreshed within the last three years; skills must have been demonstrated within previous three months

INCIDENT COMMAND SYSTEM

▷ All team members to be trained to the current ICS in operation for rope incidents.

TEAM TYPE 3 – EQUIPMENT

TRANSPORT

❭ Vehicle(s) suitable to carry personnel and equipment.

COMMUNICATIONS

❭ Handheld communications for all team members, spare batteries and charger. Waterproofed.
❭ Mobile phone with team leader and manager. Waterproofed.

NAVIGATION

❭ Handheld GPS system with street mapping facility

PPE

❭ Full PPE for all team members, plus spare:
❭ Helmet
❭ Footwear
❭ Gloves
❭ Knife
❭ Whistle
❭ Personal lighting

TECHNICAL EQUIPMENT

❭ Low stretch Kernmantle rope, minimum 100m x5
❭ Rope access equipment to allow access at height and work in suspension. This may require equipment including dynamic rope, tripod/quadpod/frame, stretcher.

ADDITIONAL EQUIPMENT

❭ Lighting
❭ Marker boards
❭ Mapping
❭ Aide-memoires
❭ Scene lighting
❭ Search lighting

MEDICAL

▷ Basic Life Support IEC (Immediate Emergency Care) Pack
▷ Oxygen cylinder x 2
▷ Resuscitation equipment
▷ Long board
▷ Blankets
▷ Basket stretcher

DECONTAMINATION

▷ Anti-bacterial hand gel
▷ Anti-bacterial face wipes
▷ Anti-bacterial equipment spray
▷ Full cleaning facilities available at base station

TESTING

▷ All equipment should be suitably tested, maintained and certified in accordance with manufacturers' guidelines.

INDIVIDUAL AND MULTI-INCIDENT FRAMEWORKS

Rescue teams, and their team leaders, may be called to individual incidents, or may be operating within a multi-incident and multi-agency framework. Team leaders should be capable of working within either situation.

Individual incidents may include a fallen hill-walker, a worker at height taken ill, or a person falling into a river. Rope Rescue Team Leaders will typically face individual incidents, rather than working within multi-incident frameworks.

Wide area flooding is the archetype of a rescuers working within a multi-agency and multi-incident framework. Water and Flood Team Leaders, in particular, need to understand the big picture. Rope Rescue Team Leaders may also face multiple incidents – eg coordinated protests.

Whilst the actual rescue techniques may remain the same, the team leader must recognise the additional impacts of multi-incident situations.

CONSIDERATIONS FOR MULTIPLE INCIDENTS

▷ Protocols for requesting additional support and/or reporting

▷ Greater demands on resources

▷ Working with partner agencies

▷ Credentialing and team typing of additional teams

▷ Increased pressure/demands from the public and media

▷ The role of the Incident Manager, and liaison between them and the Team Leader

COMMAND STRUCTURE

Gold
Strategic

The strategic (gold) level in the command structure establishes a framework to support those operating at the tactical (silver) level, by providing resources, prioritising demands, and determining plans for the return to normality.

Silver
Tactical

The tactical (silver) level in the command structure ensures that the actions taken by operational (bronze) are co-ordinated, coherent and integrated, in order to achieve maximum effectiveness and efficiency.

In a multi-agency event, silver will usually comprise the most senior officers of each agency committed with the area of operations, and will assume tactical command of the event.

Bronze
Operational

The operational (bronze) level is where the immediate work is undertaken at the emergency site(s) or other affected area.

COMMAND STRUCTURE WITH ONE OR MORE BRONZE COMMANDS

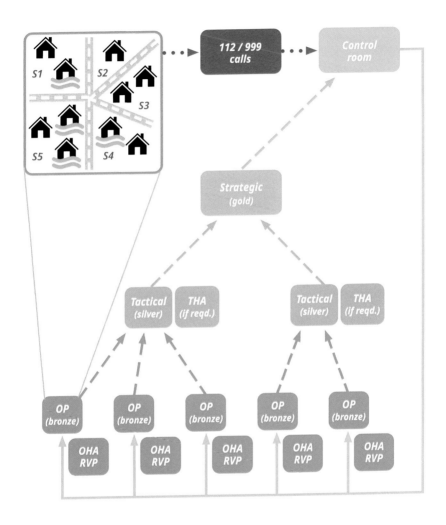

KEY

⇢⇢⇢	Command messages and resource requests
→	Mobilisation messages
•••••▶	Emergency calls
S1	Sector 1

THA = Tactical Holding Area

OHA = Operational Holding Area

RVP = Rendezvous Point

WORKING WITH PARTNER AGENCIES

▷ Who has primacy in a rescue?

▷ Where, in the incident command system (ICS) would a team operate during a rescue incident?

▷ What communication system may exist?

▷ Who do I report to?

▷ Who reports to me?

▷ What documentation would a Team Leader need to prepare and deliver?

▷ Recognition of capability, eg proof of training, ID cards.

▷ Joint training and MOUs (Memoranda of Understanding) with partner agencies.

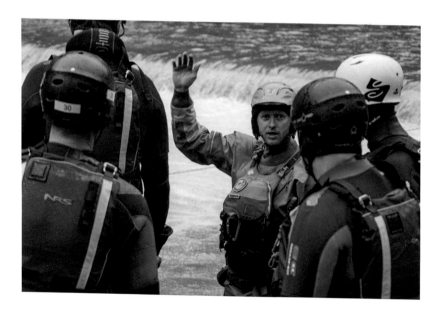

PRINCIPLES OF JOINT WORKING (JESIP)

Co-locate

Co-locate with commanders as soon as practicably possible at a single, safe and easily identified location near to the scene.

Communicate

Communicate clearly using plain language.

Co-ordinate

Co-ordinate by agreeing the lead service. Identify priorities, resources and capabilities for an effective response, including the timing of further meetings.

Jointly understand risk

Jointly understand risk by sharing information about the likelihood and potential impact of threats and hazards to agree potential control measures.

Shared situational awareness

Shared situational awareness established by using METHANE and the Joint Decision Model.

PRE-PLANNING AND RISK ASSESSMENTS

Team leaders may be directly involved in developing pre-plans, alongside training managers. In larger organisations, team leaders may have lesser involvement in developing pre-plans, but would need an awareness of existing pre-plans.

ELEMENTS OF PRE-PLANNING

▷ Management

▷ Personnel

▷ Training

▷ Experience

TYPES OF RISK ASSESSMENT

Organisations responsible for working and performing rescues in high risk environments (employers, site owners etc) must ensure that a suitable and sufficient risk assessment has been completed. They must ensure a competent person, who has the necessary skills, knowledge and experience, undertakes the risk assessment. This may be a team leader.

GENERIC RISK ASSESSMENT (GRA)

▷ Assesses the risk of an activity.

▷ Must always be in place before work.

SPECIFIC RISK ASSESSMENT (SRA)

▷ Must be in place if particular hazards exist that are not in the generic risk assessment.

▷ Site-specific, job/activity-specific or equipment-specific.

DYNAMIC RISK ASSESSMENT (DRA)

▷ On-site, real-time assessment of variables highlighted in generic/specific risk assessments.

▷ On-scene assessment of unexpected factors, environmental factors and human factors.

▷ Decision to work/not work either within remit of written risk assessments, or within competency of person performing dynamic risk assessment.

5 STAGES OF RISK ASSESSMENT

1   Identify the hazards

2   Decide who might be harmed and how

3   Evaluate the risks and decide on precautions

4   Record your findings and implement them

5   Review your assessment and update if necessary

SAMPLE RISK ASSESSMENT

Assessor:
Venue:
Has the above been assessed previously?   YES / NO

Hazard	Who might be harmed?	Risk
Look only for hazards which you could reasonably expect to result in significant harm under the routine and non-routine conditions in your workplace. Use the following examples as a guide. ▷ Slipping/tripping hazards ▷ Fire ▷ Chemicals ▷ Moving parts of machinery ▷ Work at height ▷ Ejection of material ▷ Vehicles ▷ Electricity ▷ Dust/fumes ▷ Poor lighting ▷ Low temperature ▷ Cuts ▷ Manual handling ▷ Noise	There is no need to list individuals by name. Think about groups of people who may be affected, eg: ▷ Instructors ▷ Students ▷ Members of the public Pay particular attention to: ▷ People with disabilities ▷ Young people ▷ Inexperienced staff ▷ Visitors ▷ Lone workers ▷ Pregnant/nursing women	Rate risk as high medium or low.

Date of assessment:		
Activity being assessed:		
Assessment review date:		

Existing controls	Further action	Residual risk

Have precautions already been taken against the risks from the hazards you have listed?
 	
For example:
   Adequate information, instruction or training
   Adequate systems procedures
   Adequate job safety instructions
 	
Do the precautions:
   Meet the standards set by legal requirement?
   Comply with Rescue 3 Europe standards?
   Represent good practice?
   Reduce risk as far as reasonably practicable?
 	
If so, then the risks are adequately controlled, but you need to indicate the precautions you have in place.
 	
You may refer to procedures, manuals, company rules etc.
	What more could you reasonably do for those risks which you found were not adequately controlled?
	
	Priority should be given to those risks which affect large numbers of people and/or could result in serious harm.
	
	Apply the principles below when taking further action, if possible in the following order:
	▷ Remove the risk completely
	▷ Try a less risky option
	▷ Prevent access to the hazard (eg by guarding)
	▷ Organise work to reduce exposure to the hazard
	▷ Issue personal protective equipment
		Rate risk as high, medium or low.

SAMPLE RISK ASSESSMENT, CONTINUED

Hazard	Who might be harmed?	Risk

Existing controls	Further action	Residual risk

Risk is the likelihood that a person may be harmed if exposed to a hazard.

It can be summarised as:

$$RISK = LIKELIHOOD \times SEVERITY \ (OF \ HARM)$$

'Likelihood' is the probability of a harmful event occurring, ranging from rare to almost certain.

'Severity' is a measure of the degree of harm caused, ranging from minor injury to death.

Risk can be reduced by either reducing the likelihood of harm, the severity of harm, or both.

A risk rating provides broad guidance for a course of action.

More specific/quantified scales of likelihood and severity may be used for more accurate representation of risk.

Likelihood Severity	Rare 1	Unlikely 2	Possible 3	Likely 4	Almost certain 5
Catastrophic 5	Medium	High	High	Very high	Very high
Significant 4	Medium	Medium	High	Very high	Very high
Moderate 3	Low	Medium	Medium	High	High
Low 2	Low	Low	Medium	Medium	High
Negligible 1	Low	Low	Low	Medium	Medium

HIERARCHY FOR RISK CONTROL

The ERIC-PD hierarchy for risk control has its origins in industrial workplaces, and can be used during a risk assessment.

Control measures should be selected by starting with the most effective down the least effective.

It may be necessary to select a combination of control measures, to reach an acceptable risk level.

Eliminate
> Can the risk be avoided altogether?

Replace
> Can a less hazardous technique or system be used instead?

Isolate
> Can the hazard be isolated, eg with barriers/site zoning?

Control
> Use of safe systems of work, training and supervision.

Personal Protective Equipment (PPE)
> Use of PPE, often in conjunction with risk control options above.

Discipline
> The ongoing diligence and alertness of workers/rescuers.

HUMAN FACTORS

Technical rescue systems and their components are increasingly reliable. However, humans remain fallible. Rescue systems should be designed to be tolerant of human error.

Team leaders should be aware of the ways in which human factors can influence a team's or an individual's behaviour.

Human factors can contribute to both active failures (eg an error by an operator or technician, on the ground), and latent failures (eg by decision-makers and managers, removed from front-line operations).

As the team leader is a link between operations and management, their contribution is vital in understanding human factors, causes of human failure, and assessing human reliability (the probability of successfully performing a task).

The causes of human failure can be mitigated at job/task, individual and/or organisational levels.

JOB/TASK

▷ The task should be designed in a way that matches the physical and mental limitations and strengths of the people.

INDIVIDUAL

▷ Individual strengths and weaknesses of each person.
▷ May be unchangeable (eg personality) or changeable (eg skills and attitudes).

ORGANISATIONAL

▷ Organisations must understand risk and how to mitigate accidents.
▷ Positive health and safety culture, eg risk assessment, near-miss recording systems, no-blame culture, adequate training, and undertaking operational learning.

CAUSES OF HUMAN FAILURE - ERRORS AND VIOLATIONS

Errors are unintended actions that can cause a near miss or incident. They can be categorised as slips, lapses or mistakes.

SLIP

> Doing something unplanned or incorrectly.
> Eg throwing a throwbag too late.

LAPSE

> Forgetting to do an action.
> Eg forgetting to screw up the gate of a karabiner.

MISTAKE

> Doing an action, wrongly believing it is the correct thing to do.
> Rules-based mistake - defaulting to a familiar rule or procedure, rather than accurately assessing the situation at hand.
> Knowledge- based mistake - lack of training, lack of information, or over-reliance on supposed 'experience' instead of assessing the evidence.

Violations are intended actions that can cause a near miss or incident (eg not following procedure or breaking a rule). They can be categorised as routine, situational or exceptional.

ROUTINE

> Not following the procedure has become the norm, eg lax culture.

SITUATIONAL

> The procedure isn't followed because of circumstances, eg time pressure, staffing levels, unavailable equipment etc.

EXCEPTIONAL

> In an abnormal or emergency situation, consciously deciding to break a rule in the belief that the benefit outweighs the risk.

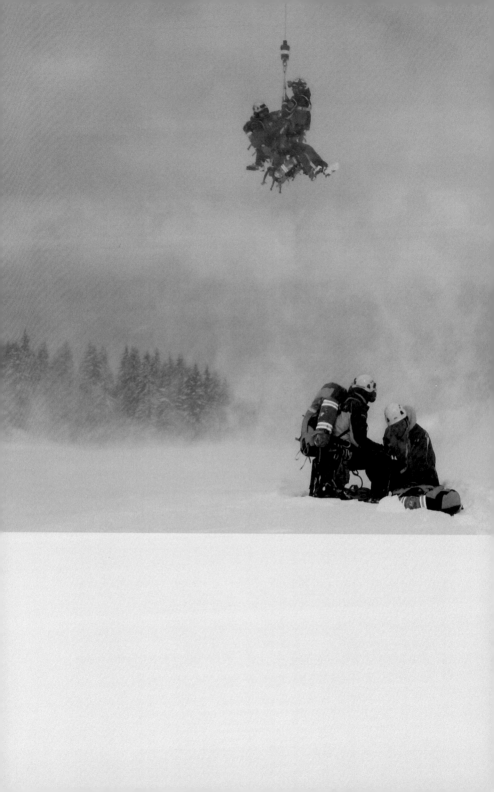

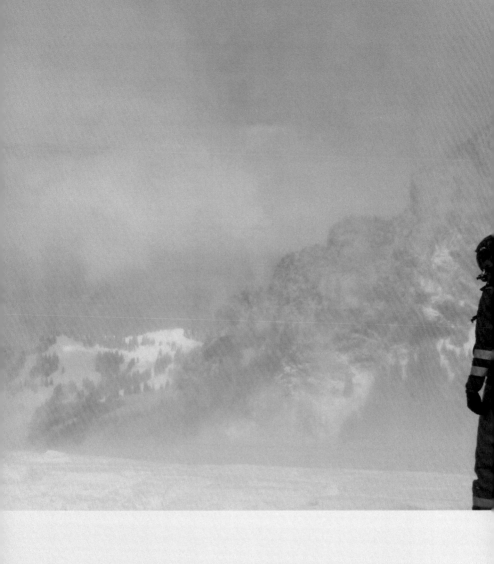

THE INCIDENT

ARRIVAL ON SCENE

STOP

Upon arrival at the rescue site, before accessing the patient, rescuers may have adrenaline pumping and feel a sense of urgency. However, they should stop and take the time to calm down and assess the situation. This will avoid mistakes being made.

CHECK

Is it safe to access the casualty? Am I going to expose myself to the same hazard as them?

Have I got everything I need to keep me safe?

Have we as a team got everything we need to keep us safe?

GO

Incident size-up and pre-deployment briefing.

The LAST principle, covering the four stages of a rescue, applies to all rescues.

Locate
> Victim
> Hazards

Access
> Difficulty level?
> Type of access - water, rope, boat, confined space, helicopter?
> Access for vehicles?
> Access for stretchers?

Stabilise
> Site containment
> Physical stabilisation - PPE?
> Medical stabilisation - ABCs? Hypothermia? Hyperthermia?

Transport
> Difficulty level? Rough terrain?
> Roped? Vertical access? Steep slopes?
> Boats? Helicopters? Landing areas?
> Nearest access for vehicles? 4x4?
> Stretchers? Number of carrying personnel

SITE ZONING

Working areas should be identified by the level of risk that they present to rescuers, support staff and bystanders. Who goes where will depend on the person's experience, training, PPE and task.

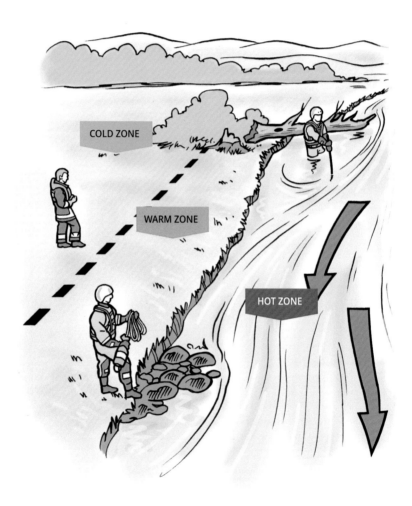

COLD ZONE

WARM ZONE

HOT ZONE

Site zoning - water

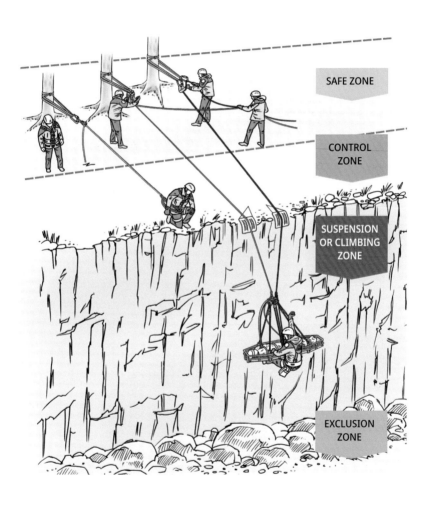

SAFE ZONE

CONTROL ZONE

SUSPENSION OR CLIMBING ZONE

EXCLUSION ZONE

Site zoning - rope

INCIDENT SIZE-UP

Upon arrival at a rescue site, a scene assessment needs to take place. This is known as size-up, and is generally much easier for locations where a pre-plan exists.

The priority is to establish what has happened, who is involved, and where, how and what the risks are.

By working through a size-up model, a team leader can establish key facts for reporting to an incident manager.

The CHALET (page 69) and M/ETHANE (page 70) size-up models can be used for incidents in all disciplines. The TEMPOE size-up model (page 71) is specifically designed for water incidents.

Team leaders should ensure that they consistently use the preferred size-up model in their locality. In the UK, for example, the Joint Emergency Services Interoperability Programme (JESIP) advocates use of the mnemonic M/ETHANE.

CHALET INCIDENT SIZE-UP MODEL

The CHALET size-up model is used for all categories of incident, including water, rope, boat, confined space and ice rescue.

Casualties

Numbers of casualties? Adults/children? Fatalities? Medical resources required?

Hazards

Physical eg loose rock? Environmental eg weather? Bystanders? Industrial hazmat?

Access

How easy to access rescue site? How easy is onward transportation of casualty? Nearest vehicle access?

Location

OS grid reference or GPS latitude and longitude. Local name. What3Words.

Emergency services

Fire/police/ambulance? Mountain/lowland rescue? Helicopter? Animal rescue? Which are on-scene and who else is required?

Type of incident

Major incident?
Water examples – Vehicle in water? Kayak pin?
Rope examples – Fall? Stranded victim(s)?

M/ETHANE INCIDENT SIZE-UP MODEL

The M/ETHANE size-up model is used for all categories of incident, including water, rope, boat, confined space and ice rescue.

My call sign/Major incident declared

Exact location

OS grid reference or GPS latitude and longitude. Local name. What3Words.

Type of incident

Major incident?
Water examples – Vehicle in water? Kayak pin?
Rope examples – Fall? Stranded victim(s)?

Hazards, present and potential

Physical eg loose rock? Environmental eg weather? Bystanders? Industrial hazmat?

Access and egress

How easy to access rescue site? How easy is onward transportation of casualty? Nearest vehicle access?

Number and severity of casualties

Numbers of casualties? Adults/children? Fatalities? Medical resources required?

Emergency services

Fire/police/ambulance? Mountain/lowland rescue? Helicopter? Animal rescue? Which are on-scene and who else is required?

TEMPOE WATER INCIDENT SIZE-UP MODEL

The TEMPOE size-up model is designed for water rescue incidents.

Time and temperature

Time incident occurred. Arrival on scene. Submersion/immersion duration. Time-critical casualties? Victim capabilities. Rescue or body recovery?

Energy and equipment

Energy of water – high or low? What resources are available now? Are the resources suitable for energy level and conditions? What resources are available later? When?

Movement and measurement

Water level – rising or falling? Weather impacts. Upstream spotters. Appropriate downstream containment in place? True rescue? Known mobile victim? Static victim?

Personnel and plan

Identify priorities. Set clear objectives and record in decision log. Consider rescue options (LAST). Sufficient trained people? Appropriate equipment? Call in additional teams or resources (including other agencies). Plan B? Plan C? Rendezvous point (RVP) and approach route. Brief teams.

Operate

Dynamic risk assessment. Is the incident changing? Constant evaluation of tactics/system of work. Do not be afraid to change tactics/system of work if necessary.

Evaluate

Ongoing evaluation. Post-incident evaluation.

DECISION-MAKING MODELS

After sizing-up the incident, the team leader must select a course of action. Decision-making models can assist in this process, such as JESIP's Joint Decision-Making Model, and the 5+2 Model used extensively in Switzerland.

The Joint Decision-Making Model may be overseen by managers, drawing on information from team leaders. The 5+2 Model is designed for use by team leaders on the ground.

MULTI-AGENCY DECISION-MAKING MODEL

THE JOINT DECISION-MAKING MODEL (JESIP)

The JESIP Joint Decision-Making Model is used by incident managers, identifying and communicating the 'what', 'when' and 'who' of their strategy.

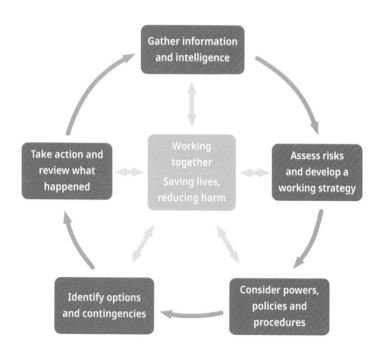

The information supplied by team leaders feeds into the multi-agency joint decision-making process.

INCIDENT LOCATION

INCIDENT TYPE

INFORMATION AND INTELLIGENCE

THREATS, RISKS AND WORKING STRATEGY

POWERS, POLICIES AND PROCEDURES

OPTIONS AND CONTINGENCIES

ACTIONS REQUIRED

NEXT REVIEW

TEAM LEADER DECISION-MAKING MODEL

THE 5+2 MODEL

The 5+2 model is widely used by the military and emergency services in Switzerland to assist their team leaders to size-up and make decisions on how to deal with an incident. The model here is adapted, with permission, from IPH, the Interkantonale Polizeischule Hitzkirch.

The 5 refers the 5 phases that team leaders need to consider before making a decision. The 2 refers to any immediate actions required, and time factors during the incident.

Whilst the 5 points are generally worked through in order, the 2 points about immediate actions and time factors are constantly reviewed to ensure that the plan of action being decided on by the team leader is still the best course of action. If changes are identified, they can then be implemented.

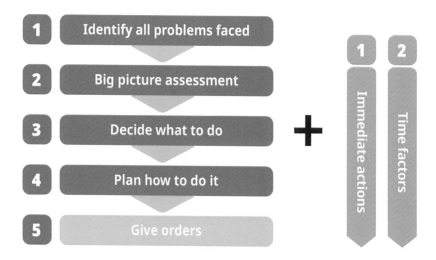

1. Identify all problems faced
2. Big picture assessment
3. Decide what to do
4. Plan how to do it
5. Give orders

+

1. Immediate actions
2. Time factors

Identify all problems faced

Type of incident

Number of casualties

Access and egress issues

?

Equipment and personnel needed

Hazards

Specialist equipment needed

2   Big picture assessment

The team leader should keep an overview of the whole incident and the 'big picture' at all times. They should monitor for changes as the incident progresses, such as river levels, weather, available light, so that any necessary changes can be implemented.

By reviewing the task at hand, the time available, the nature of the incident and the environment the team is working in, a decision can be made on what needs to be done.

The big picture should be communicated to all team members, so that they have an understanding of what the team is trying to achieve, even if they end up working in isolation.

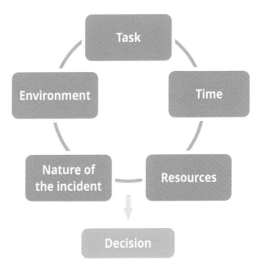

3   Decide what to do

Before deployment, the team leader needs to decide on a course of action, and which techniques are most appropriate, based on the information in stages 1 and 2.

4   Plan how to do it

Once a decision has been made as to the course of action, the team leader can plan how best to conduct the rescue. Are the site, personnel and equipment suitable for the chosen technique? Eg, in a water rescue where boat on a highline has been identified as an appropriate rescue technique, are there the anchors, conditions and trained personnel to set up and work the system? These decisions are made based on information from the prior steps and a site analysis.

5   Give orders

The team leader should inform the team of the course of action, ensuring that the team understands and has the training to carry out the task.

The orders given by the team leader can be broken down into 5 subcategories: Orientation, Intention, Assignments, Special Orders and Locations - see right.

Constant review of big picture

At all times it is essential to monitor the big picture, to ensure that there have been no changes or developments that affect what a team leader and the rescue team are doing.

5 cont. Give orders - subcategories

A

Orientation
Incident, location and possible development of the situation.
Team's own assignment and structure of the task.
Additional support (partner agencies).

B

Intention *(verbalised decision)*
Detailed briefing of how, with what resources, and in what chronological order, the plan is to be fulfilled.
Defines solutions to subproblems that were identified in the size-up.

C

Assignments
Assigning team members, and their resources, to specific tasks.

D

Special orders
Additional tactical, technical and/or logistical instructions.
May be for the whole team, or an individual.
Communication. Time planning. Emergency procedures. Catering.
Equipment. Anything else?

E

Locations
Team leader's own location.
Command locations of the operations manager and third parties.

TEAM BRIEFING

Team leaders should ensure that they consistently use the preferred team briefing model in their locality.

Models presented here include a pre-rig/pre-deployment model used in rope and confined space rescues (page 79), GSMEAC (page 80) and IIMARCH (page 82) which are used for rescues in all disciplines, STAR (page 84) which is often used in industrial environments, and Big Picture REDO (page 85), which is often used in rope and confined space rescues.

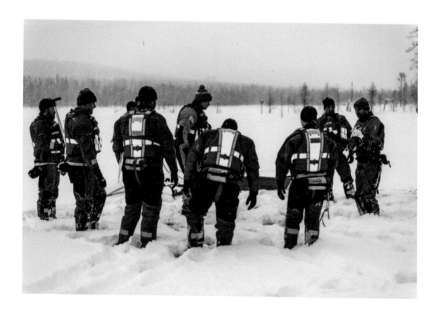

PRE-RIG/PRE-DEPLOYMENT BRIEFING

The pre-rig briefing model is generally used in rope and confined space incidents, but can be adapted to a pre-deployment briefing model for water, boat, ice and confined space incidents.

WHAT WE FACE

WHAT WE ARE GOING TO DO

WHY WE ARE GOING TO DO THAT

HAZARDS

> **Now talk to me...**
> *(Does anybody see anything I've missed or have a better idea?)*

The team leader should reiterate that:

Anyone can call STOP if they have safety concerns!

GSMEAC BRIEFING MODEL

The GSMEAC briefing model creates a structured format for a briefing. It originated in the military, but can be used by rescue team leaders for water, rope, boat, confined space and ice incidents.

Ground (optional)

> Description of geography

Situation

> General information
> Weather details
> Location details
> Infrastructure

Mission

> Outline of objectives.
> Detailed objectives.

Execution

> Detailed description of how the objectives are going to be achieved.
> Detailed roles for individual team members.
> Health and safety briefing
> Plan for emerging volunteers
> Brief to conclusion – eg where to take casualties and when to return to holding area, if applicable.

Administration

> Continued monitoring and recording of information.
> Any pre-planning already activated.
> Command Support needed and where
> Logging of decisions and events
> Sit reps frequency
> Information sharing
> Navigation, mapping, local guides
> Relief teams
> Where credentialing will take place (if necessary)
> Welfare

A

Command, control and communications

> Command structure
> Roles of other agencies
> Communications structure, call signs etc.
> Exit from incident procedure

C

Any questions?

IIMARCH BRIEFING MODEL

The IIMARCH briefing model is commonly used by UK emergency services operating under the Joint Emergency Services Interoperability Programme (JESIP).

Information
> What, where, when, how, how many, so what, what might?
> Timeline and history (if applicable).

Intent
> Why are we here?
> What are we trying to achieve?

Method
> How are we going to do it?

Administration

> What is required for effective, efficient and safe implementation?
> Identification of:
  - Commanders.
  - Tasking.
  - Timing.
  - Decision logs.
  - Equipment.
  - Dress code.
  - PPE.
  - Welfare.
  - Food.
  - Logistics.

Risk assessment

> What are the relevant risks?
> What measures are required to mitigate them?

Communications

> How are we going to initiate and maintain communications with all partners and interested parties?

Humanitarian issues

> What humanitarian assistance and human rights issues arise or may arise from this event and the response to it?

STAR BRIEFING MODEL

The STAR briefing model has its origins in industrial environments, including work at height and work in confined space.

Site

> Location
> Nature of site
> Hazards/risks and control measures
> Access/egress
> Zones

Task

> Description of the task

Actions

> Team roles
> Communications
> Equipment/resources required
> Welfare arrangements

Rescue/emergency arrangements

> Actions in the event of an incident/emergency that exceeds the rescue team's capability

BIG PICTURE REDO BRIEFING MODEL

The Big Picture REDO briefing model is generally used by rope and confined space rescue teams.

Big picture

> Enhances situational awareness.
> Ensures different agencies are aware of each other (including over radio).
> Significant hazards are identified.
> Enables latecomers to understand what is expected.

Roll call

> Focuses attention.
> Allows last-minute adjustments.

Edge transition brief

> Establishes the methodology.

Dry run

> Establishes a common mental model of the operation with all participants.

Operate

> Make a clear distinction between the dry run and the go-live phase.

TEAM WELFARE

The team leader may be directly responsible for team welfare, or a separate welfare officer may be appointed.

Welfare is an important issue in all rescue environments. Working in harsh environments can quickly take its toll on people.

It is important to:

▷ Take regular breaks.

▷ Rotate teams.

▷ Ensure sufficient food, water, shelter and welfare facilities are available for all rescuers.

Welfare considerations may be defined within team typing and/or operational guidance. They include:

▷ Basic medical screening to ensure appropriate levels of fitness

▷ Food and drink

▷ Bathroom/toilet breaks and facilities

▷ Temporary shelters

▷ Deployment times and suitable rest breaks

▷ Rotation of team members where necessary

▷ Medical and decontamination facilities

▷ Accommodation for long deployments

▷ Post-incident debriefing (page 92)

▷ Mental health considerations (page 97)

MEDIA CONSIDERATIONS

Team leaders should refer media requests to the incident manager and/or their organisation's media team.

My official media liaison is:
Their contact details are: **Phone:** **Mobile:** **Email:** **Other:**

Team leaders must be mindful of public and media impressions of their actions. They must brief their team about these considerations.

The messages used by managers and media teams are likely to use pre-planned statements, which use language appropriate to the incident, to prevent undue alarm or speculation.

If a team leader is asked to support an incident manager or media team during an interview, there are some key interview considerations.

▷ Ensure permission has been granted for the interview.

▷ Agree suitable location, ie not in area of risk.

▷ Pre-plan appropriate community safety or corporate messages.

▷ Be aware of topics or information that should not be communicated publicly.

▷ Check latest situation from Control prior to interview.

▷ Wear appropriate uniform, PPE and headwear for location.

▷ Express sympathy for those affected by the incident.

▷ Do not comment on other agencies unless to praise when appropriate.

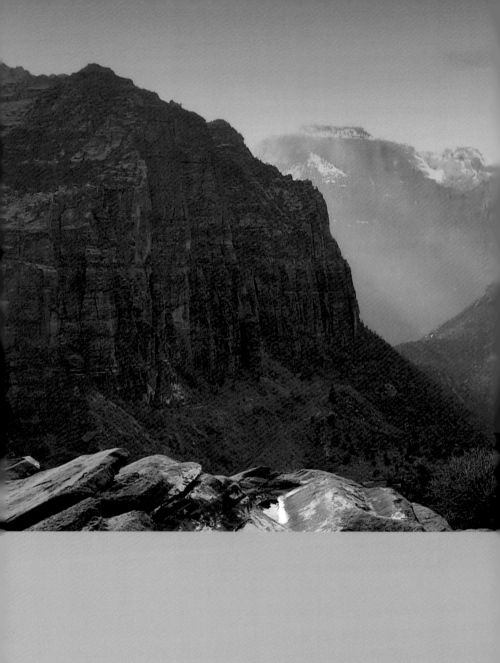

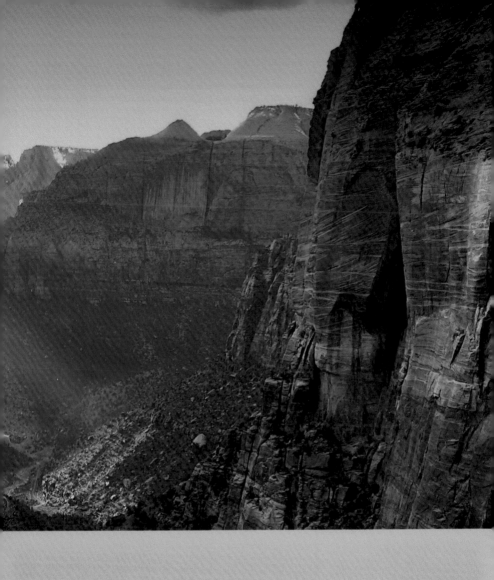

POST-INCIDENT

PATIENT HANDOVER

The ATMIST patient handover tool can be used when passing a casualty to a medical team.

Age
> Also include other details of casualty, eg casualty's name and gender.

Time
> Time of incident.
> Estimated time of arrival at handover.

Mechanism
> Key mechanism of incident injury (eg drowning, falling).
> Other factors associated with major injuries.

Injuries
> Injuries from top to toe.
> Seen injuries.
> Suspected injuries.

Signs
> First set of vital signs of patient.
> Changes to vital signs? Improvement or deterioration?

Treatment
> Treatment given to the casualty.

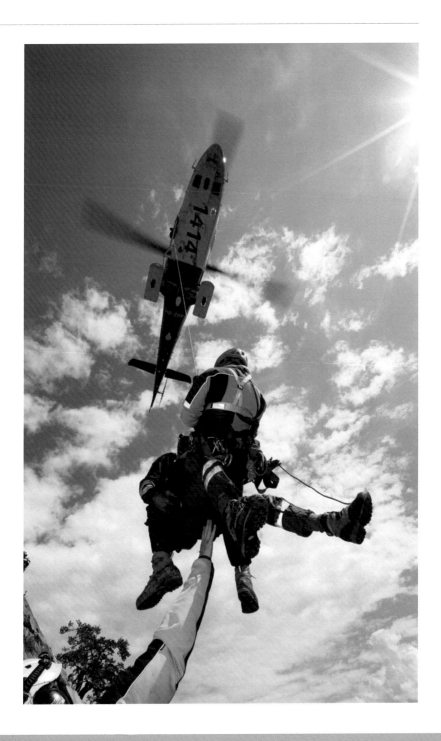

DEBRIEFING

Following an incident, the team leader should debrief their team. This may be a 'hot' debrief talking to rescuers at the scene, and/or a more formal operational debrief, eg back at base.

Debriefings should be recorded. Using a structured format allows the team leader to capture the relevant information from the incident, to report up the chain of command, enabling lessons to be learned and follow-up actions to be applied.

RESCUER WELFARE

Including immediate physical and mental health concerns during hot debrief.

WHAT HAPPENED?

Brief synopsis, and chronology where applicable.

PPE AND EQUIPMENT

Did all PPE and equipment function correctly?
Anything to be isolated, checked and potentially retired?

TRAINING LEVEL

Was the training level of all rescuers sufficient?

POLICIES

Were the organisation's relevant policies appropriate, or are there suggestions for improvement?

AREAS FOR IMPROVEMENT

What could have been done differently or better?

FUTURE ACTIONS

What next?

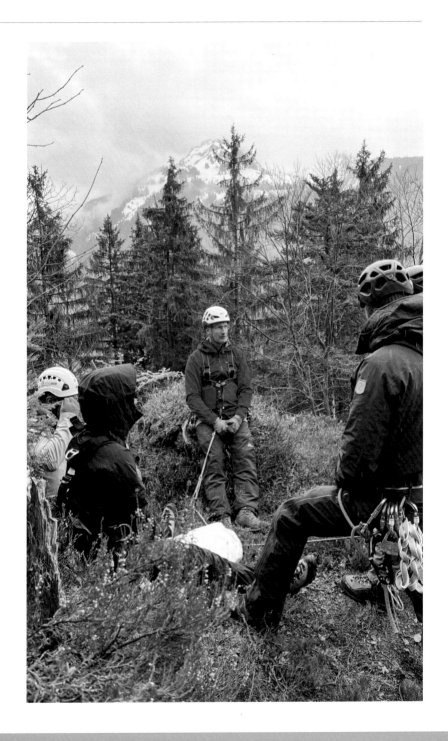

POST-INCIDENT PROCEDURES, PAPERWORK AND REPORTING

▷ Handover of responsibility

▷ Search areas and times where appropriate

▷ Medical considerations and accident reporting

▷ Chain of command and reporting procedure

▷ Closing down of an incident

INCIDENT REPORT FORMS

An example of an incident report form is on pages 95-96. Organisations may choose to use their own format, but the key information within them should be universal. Team leaders may need to complete incident report forms.

Risk assessments (page 52) should also be reviewed after an incident.

ABOUT YOU

What is your full name?

What is your job title?

What is your telephone number?

ABOUT YOUR ORGANISATION

What is the name of your organisation?

What is the address and postcode?

ABOUT THE AFFECTED PERSON

What is their full name?

What is their home address and postcode?

How old are they?

Was the affected person:
☐ An employee
☐ A member of the public
☐ Other (please describe)

ABOUT THE INCIDENT

Was the incident:
☐ A fatality
☐ A major injury
☐ An injury leading to more than 3 days off work
☐ An injury leading to 0–2 days off work
☐ A near miss
☐ Other (please describe)

Did the affected person
☐ Become unconscious
☐ Need resuscitation
☐ Remain in hospital for more than 24 hours
☐ None of the above

On what date did the incident happen?

At what time did the incident happen?

What were the environmental conditions like? Eg water levels, weather conditions.

ATTACHMENTS

Additional sheets attached? Eg photos, continuation sheets.
☐ Yes   ☐ No

REPORTING AN INJURY, DANGEROUS OCCURRENCE OR NEAR MISS

LOCATION

Where did the incident happen?
Use, eg, grid reference, local names for stretch of river or training venue, and/or draw map

N

ABOUT THE INCIDENT

Describe in as much detail as you can what happened. If it was a personal injury, describe what the person was doing. Use extra sheets if necessary.

Signature	Date

Rescue team leaders and team members should be aware of their own and their colleagues' mental health, particularly following an unsuccessful or traumatic rescue attempt. The International Society for Traumatic Stress Studies identifies a number of negative outcomes as a result of occupational trauma exposure (below).

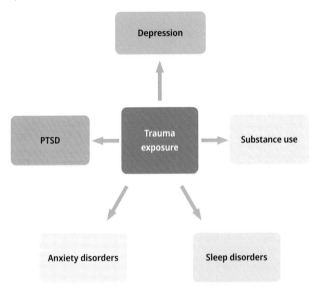

Thankfully, the stigma of talking about mental health issues and seeking help is less than it once was. However, there is still much work to be done to achieve understanding and acceptance from everyone.

Modern and forward-thinking organisations may have access to mental health support and therapy for rescuers, or there may be access through rescuers' unions, or charity organisations.

In the UK, for example, mental health charity Mind have put together a toolkit called Our Frontline, which offers free resources, links and contacts. See https://www.mentalhealthatwork.org.uk/toolkit/ourfrontline-emergency/